Essential Oils

Top 50 Essential Oils and Aromatherapy DIY Recipes For Stress Relief, Relaxation And Better Sleep

JANE WOLFE

Copyright © 2017 by Jane Wolfe

Table of Contents

Introduction

I want to thank you and congratulate you for downloading the book, *"Essential Oils: Top 50 Essential Oils and Aromatherapy DIY Recipes For Stress Relief, Relaxation And Better Sleep"*.

This book has actionable information on how to use essential oils to fight stress, get better sleep and enhance relaxation.

Today, use of essential oils has become common thanks to general communal understanding of their physical health benefits. However, and as unfortunate as this sounds, although currently gaining wide use and acceptance, very few actually understand the entire scope of the healing capabilities of essential oils.

That notwithstanding, most of us know about the everyday power of scent. For instance, we know that a particular perfume can remind you of your beloved while the smell of your favorite body spray can rekindle memories of your first date or particular anniversary. Whichever the case, scents or aroma can greatly influence various areas of your life including health and general wellbeing. In particular, aromas from essential oils can help you relax, fight stress, sleep better, or improve your sex life!

This book vividly discusses the physical and emotional benefits of essential oils and by so doing, creates a user-friendly essential oil guide that shall show you how to use essential oils to take charge of your emotional health.

By reading this book, you will gain a breath of knowledge that shall help you use essential oils like a pro and start appreciating their distinct healing qualities. Written to cater to long-time oil enthusiasts as well as beginners, this guidebook will inspire you to use the genius as well as beauty of Mother Nature's finest gifts, essential oils, to foster optimal personal health.

Let's begin.

Thanks again for downloading this book. I hope you enjoy it!

Let's begin by answering the question, "what are essential oils" in the simplest manner possible and then move on to discussing why oils are important to you and how to use them.

An Introduction To Essential Oils

What are Essential Oils?

Essential oils are fragrant, highly concentrated natural compounds that come from various parts of plants such as flowers, roots, bark, stems, and seeds. These oils are also known as volatile oils or ethereal oils, and are responsible for the distinctive smell in some plants.

The oils are generally non-water based phytochemicals constituted of aromatic compounds. They are generally pure, crisp to the touch, and quickly absorbed by the skin, which is why their most common application is topical application or through massage.

Most essential oils range from clear to deep blue in color in their pure and unmodified (commonly referred to as unadulterated) form. As compared to other oils, essential oils are fat-soluble but lack the fatty acids or lipids ordinarily found in vegetable and animal oils.

Closely related to essential oils are perfumes. At their most basic form, perfumes are aromatic or sweet smelling, which is why many users confuse perfumes and essential. The fact of the matter, however, is that essential oils are not kin to "fragrance oils" or body perfumes since the former comes from true plants. On the contrary, perfumes are artificial creations that often contain artificial ingredients that do not offer the therapeutic benefits offered by essential oils.

The purity of essential oils and method of extraction from parent plant matters a lot. Essential oils or "natural oils from plants" do not undergo any chemical processing. For this reason, the oils do not undergo any modification that alters their chemical constituents and are likely to offer the full benefits intended.

Talking of benefits, we need to discuss how essential oils actually influence your body and mind. Simply put, we need to discuss why, to relieve stress, you should massage aromatic oils onto your skin instead of reaching for prescription drugs such as antidepressants.

First, and as opposed to pharmaceutical medications, essential oils are natural compounds and when used correctly, they minimize, to a margin of zero, the chances of undesirable side effects. Secondly, essential oils are just as, and at times more effective than, their pharmaceutical counterparts. The effectiveness of essential oils depends on the active ingredients present in the oil as well as how these ingredients interact with your body and mind.

Before we discuss the distinct properties of essential oils responsible for the various benefits, let us first see how oils affect you.

How Essential Oils Affect Your Body

Natural oils from plants have the potential to affect your body, mind, and emotions mainly because of the presence of various compounds. Depending on the method of application, these compounds directly interact with various body parts such as the skin and lungs.

For instance, once you inhale essential oils, the aroma molecules pass through the olfactory membrane that forms the nasal lining. These molecules stimulate the nerve cells to generate electrical impulses sent to the olfactory bulb located in your brain. This bulb transmits the electrical signals to the amygdala, the part of the brain responsible for storing emotional memories.

Apart from the amygdala, the electrical impulses also reach other limbic parts of the brain such as the limbic lobe comprised of the hippocampus, a system that has a direct link to the part of the brain that controls memory, breathing, heart rate, and hormonal balance and stress levels.

Because of how these aromas influence the limbic system, essential oils can induce positive psychological and physiological effects on your mind and body. For instance, the olfactory nerves respond to aromas by telling your brain to produce neurochemicals and hormones. Research has shown that these byproducts have the potential to alter your psychology in various ways. How does this happen, you may ask? Well, the aroma from essential oils stimulates the limbic system, a system that has a direct activating impact on the hypothalamus. As far as *altering your psychology* is concerned, this is the initial point. Let us understand psychology:

For starters, psychology refers to the study of the human mind as well as its functions and in particular regarding those, which that affect behavior in a particular context. In relation to the link between psychology and hypothalamus, the hypothalamus is a gland that produces hormones that control all bodily functions, hormones such as the thyroid hormones, sex hormones, and growth hormones. Furthermore, it releases neurotransmitters such as serotonin that controls other processes such as pain control, sleep cycle, and immune function.

As already stated, the fragrance or aroma in essential oils directly influences the hypothalamus and limbic lobe of the brain. Therefore, each inhalation of oil can effectively stimulate these brain regions to relieve emotional problems such as stress and trauma. In so doing, essential oils work in a manner similar manner to how most sedatives or antidepressants work.

For these reasons, essential oils are applicable in various disciplines such as medicine and alternative healing in what we refer to as *aromatherapy*, the practice of utilizing the natural oils extracted from plants to improve physical and psychological wellbeing.

At this point, you may be wondering what makes essential oils so important? Is there any specific active ingredient in these oils that largely affects your body, mind, or brain and makes them such powerful healing agents?

Let us see just how therapeutic and beneficial essential oils are and look at the explanation behind their effectiveness, as the benefits largely depend on the properties.

The Benefits of Essential Oils

Here is a detailed list of a few benefits you can derive from using unprocessed or unadulterated essential oils:

1: Fight Stress

Worrying about the never-ending demands of life can negatively affect your emotional health especially if the stress is uncontrollable. If you are already struggling with stress, you need to start using essential oils to get relief since research has proven that essential oils are great chronic stress remedies.

How do they do that?

Well, the scents produced by specific essential oils stimulate the central nervous system, the system that controls emotion. The limbic system produces beneficial chemicals such as serotonin and endorphin, hormones that have a great influence on the central nervous system. Serotonin helps combat stress and anxiety; on the other hand, endorphins are soothing to pain and can boost your happiness.

2: Promote Relaxation

Relaxation is the state of being free from tension and anxiety. Research has shown that after a hectic day, essential oils can boost energy levels in the same way as meditation or exercising.

While both practices promote relaxation, you can "effortlessly" adopt aromatherapy to stimulate your physical, emotional, and psychological being. Essential oils work by stimulating your body and mind, and boosting blood circulation, which helps promote relaxation.

The most recommended way to use essential oils to promote relaxation is to do an *aroma-therapeutic bath*. Just add 5-10 drops of your favorite essential oil (of course you use those essential oils that help fulfill this purpose) into a bathtub to turn a routine bath into a refreshing experience.

Note: Do not add essential oils to running water because doing so may lead to evaporation, which may reduce efficiency.

3: Facilitates Sleep

"Sleep deprivation" can be a very dangerous problem that makes you "groggy" or tired, and can cripple you on a physical, mental, emotional, and social level. In fact, not getting enough sleep can cause side effects such as increased irritability, mood imbalance, caffeine addiction, difficult concentrating, and in some cases, nerve dysfunction. While many people use over-the-counter drugs to enhance sleep, these can have undesirable side effects like making you to be overly dependent on them. The good news is that you can adopt natural remedies that have no possible addictions or undesired side effects.

Since essential oils can easily penetrate the skin (transdermal), topically massaging the oils on the skin is a very effective way to treat sleep disorders. Oils such as lavender can enter the blood stream within 5 minutes of body massage and within 20 minutes, we can observe a maximum concentration level of the oil.

Additional studies suggest that aromatherapy can restore sleep quality and duration better than benzodiazepines, particularly in older people. In fact, lavender essential oil offers effective temporary relief from continued use of pharmaceutical sleep aids and can greatly reduce side effects of drugs.

Note:

1. To achieve these benefits, you need to obtain genuine, pure, and authentic essential oils as opposed to adulterated varieties that may lead to adverse reactions. For instance, if used on a plant before the extraction of an essential oil, substances such as chemicals and pesticides can negatively affect the quality of essential oils.

2. Also, be aware that in some cases, oil-manufacturing companies can over-distil essential oils, dilute them, or chemically alter the quality of therapeutic oils. This makes the oils of lower quality, less valuable, and thus unsuitable for home or clinical application. To understand how to choose oils, avoid essential oil products that tend to be sweet or edible because they are often over-processed.

3. Further, if not improperly packaged or handled, exposure to oxygen, heat, or light can adversely compromise the quality and effectiveness of an essential oil. For instance, oils from citrus fruits are likely to undergo oxidation, a process that alters their chemical composition. This means when you use oxidized citrus fruits oils, you will not derive the much need benefits.

4. When buying essential oils for home or commercial use, only buy 100% pure *therapeutic-grade* essential oils; such oils meet the required distillation standards and do not include solvents such as water or other oils. In addition, get into the habit of reading labels so you can differentiate pure oils from blends based on the list of constituents.

Once you have taken all the precautionary measures, you can start using essential oils for various applications. Here, the rule of thumb is to know how to adopt aromatherapy or use of essential oils, and the simple guidelines you should observe. If you understand the basics, applying an essential oil should not be a complicated process. Essentially, the method of application depends on the type of oil under use or the condition you want to treat.

In the next section, we shall discuss simple ways to use essential oils:

Various Ways to Use Essential Oils

You can apply essential oils in different ways to derive different benefits. With that said, the most common application methods include inhaling and topical application to the skin. Let us discuss how each works:

1: Inhalation

To fight stress, nausea, or fatigue symptoms, you can directly inhale essential oils such as eucalyptus or peppermint. As I already stated, when you inhale these oils, the airborne molecules in oils interact with the olfactory and respiratory systems through the lungs and the limbic system of the brain linked to emotions.

For starters, inhaling therapeutic oils is dummy-simple! All you need to do is heat water in a small bowl, add a few drops of your favorite essential oils, and then breathe in the generated stream.

Alternatively, dab 1-3 drops of your favorite oil on a tissue or cotton ball, position it near your nose, and inhale. When doing the initial inhale, try a single drop of diluted oil to check for sensitivity to the oil.

Furthermore, you can inhale fumes from an essential oil burner.

2: Skin Application

Some oils work best when applied on the skin, the largest organ in the body and in so doing, bring about a wide array of benefits. For instance, when applied to the skin, essential oils such as ginger, black pepper oil, and related blends can help reduce arthritis pain and boost flexibility.

Such oils are particularly helpful to the skin as they easily seep into the cells of hair follicles. Your skin is permeable to the active chemicals found in essential oils. These active ingredients work in a manner similar to the working modalities of topical creams or nicotine patches resulting to various benefits. For instance, the oils reach your sebaceous glands where they combine with the natural moisturizers thus enhancing the supple nature of the skin.

The easiest and most effective way to apply essential oils on the skin or topically is through body massage, as body massage can greatly increase absorption of essential oils given that massaging essential oils on the skin boosts blood circulation in stimulated areas. To massage, simply rub and press the essential oil or its blend on various points of your skin or face, taking care not to affect your eyes. Rub on the side of each nostril, across the forehead, inside the eyebrows, and on the temples.

Note: Essential oils absorb faster where there is greater concentration of hair follicles and sweat glands. This therefore means you should apply your chosen essential oil on areas such as the armpits, palms, soles, head, and genitals. Make sure to dilute the essential oils before use though.

3: Bathing

Commonly called *hydrotherapy,* ordinary bathing can be a form of natural medicine. In hydrotherapy, we use water at different temperatures to stimulate various systems of the body. For instance, various methods of hydrotherapy procedures such as winter swimming can help lower fatigue and tension, boost mood, and relieve pain. You can introduce the use of essential oils in hydrotherapy to bring about unique benefits of essential oils in hydrotherapy. For instance, if you suffer from painful conditions such as rheumatism, asthma, or fibromyalgia, water therapy with essential oils can better your general wellbeing.

To incorporate oils into your bath, simply add around 10 drops of the oil to your bath water and then soak in the water to allow the skin enough time to absorb the elements in the oil. When bathing with essential oils, you kill two birds with one stone in that you also inhale the vapor released by the oils!

As you bathe in essential oils, consider adding the essential oils just before you get into bath; otherwise the volatile oil may evaporate if left in water. Additionally, consider the kind of scented oils you add to your bath water; essential oils such as lemon, clove, eucalyptus, aniseed, peppermint, spearmint, and orange can sting. Therefore, to avoid counter reactivity or possible skin burns, only use a few drops of your favorite oil.

Talking of "skin burns" and other related problems, here is what you should know about the safe use of essential oils:

Essential Oil Safety Usage

Although essential oils have therapeutic or healing properties, they can lead to contraindication especially if a user suffers from allergies, epilepsy, or blood pressure problems. For instance, in an instance where you are allergic to some of the elements in an essential oil, the skin may develop hives or itchy rashes.

However, as long as you follow the recommended safety rules, everything should go well. One of the simplest rules is never attempt to use essential oil on inflamed, diseased, or damaged skin. This rule helps prevent an adverse reaction.

Generally, the safe use of essential oils depends on factors such as:

Dilution Level

Essential oils are *concentrated* compounds; this means before you use them, the first thing you should do is dilute them in vegetable oils such as almond, avocado, or jojoba oil.

The recommended dilution level is about 1-5 percent, i.e. up to 95 percent of vegetable oil (also called carrier oil) diluting 5 percent essential oil. The rule of thumb here is never to inhale or use massage essential oils that have a higher concentration of more than 5 percent as this may lead to skin reactions or skin burns.

Moreover, keep in mind that that prolonged exposure to highly concentrated oils can lead to undesired effects like nausea, headaches, convulsions, and lethargy.

For pregnant women, you can only use essential oils in your first trimester and in mild concentrations; the best way to use essential oils during pregnancy is to dilute them to 1 percent, but it is advisable to avoid them altogether if you have a history of miscarriages. Throughout your pregnancy, avoid most of the oils apart from lavender, tangerine, and Neroli.

Application Methods

Not all oils can be used using the same method since oils meant for inhalation may pose a health risk if applied topically on the skin. For instance, oils like cinnamon, thyme, clove, and oregano are sometimes suitable for inhalation as can cause skin irritation if massaged on skin.

Moreover, others like citrus fruit essential oils react with the skin when exposed to the sun. Thus, after applying citrus fruit oils such as lemon, orange, or bergamot, do not expose your skin to ultra-violet light. Such oils are extremely photosensitive and exposure to sunlight or sun-bed radiation immediately after their application can result in severe skin burns.

Another thing: never eat or ingest essential oils unless instructed to do so by a qualified aromatherapist. This is because essential oils are concentrated and contain active compounds that can directly damage internal organs. The most recommended application methods are massage, inhalation, and hydrotherapy.

That's not all; while massaging oils on your skin, do not apply oils near your eyes or mucous membranes to prevent possible reactions.

The Dosage

Using essential oils in wrong dosages or extremely high concentrations can lead to negative outcomes such as the growth of tumorous cells. Moreover, wrong dosage of oils can damage the skin if applied topically, and the liver if inhaled in higher than recommended dosages.

You should dilute oils as dictated by the recipe or application to avoid possible contraindications.

Note: Be aware that young children, toddlers, and infants are likely to be over sensitive to strong essential oils. For them, the safe dilution level should be about 0.5-2.5 percent, which mainly depends on the condition addressed.

Purity

Some companies are likely to modify or adulterate oils by combining them with synthetic chemicals in a bid to improve scent or shelf life. Some essential oil production companies may also dilute some essential oil brands with vegetable oils to over 50 percent. Compared to pure oils, such oils may not give you similar results.

Oils such as rose or Neroli are the oils commonly affected by over-dilution by companies with the aim of lowering production costs. Therefore, when buying these oils, take extra care.

How can you do so bearing in mind that the labeling may not suggest the dilution or purity level? Well, the truth is that it is hard to detect overly diluted or adulterated oils. Nonetheless, there are a few ways to segregate genuine essential oil products from the lot of fake ones. One thing is that overly processed oils tend to be sweeter or "edible" because of the synthetic additives or processing methods used to produce them. What is worse about processing essential oils is that high heat can also denature the active agents in such oils.

To avoid buying "cheap oils," watch out for bottles labeled as "perfume oils" or "fragrance oils" as these are very different from essential oils. Also important to note is that you need to go for essential oils sold in small and colored bottles as the packing of fake products is often in very big and clear bottles. Therapeutic oils also come in smaller bottles because of the initial cost of producing an ounce of high quality oil. Conduct internet research on the recommended retail prices for high quality oils so that you can easily tell those that look too cheap.

Let's discuss the storage and handling of essential oils next:

Storage and Handling of Essential Oils

Factors such as packaging, handling, and storage can lower the quality of essential oils especially if exposed to heat, oxygen, and light. For instance, oils from the citrus family like lime and lemon are likely to oxidize when exposed to the environment. Therefore, for citrus oils, store them in a refrigerator between 5-10 degrees Celsius to avoid damage or oxidation from temperature variations.

Some oils are volatile; thus, replace the cap after each use. Further, to avoid chemical breakdown, store such oils in well-closed and dark bottles away from heat or direct light. Moreover, consider writing down the date you first opened the bottle given that the quality of essential oils reduces over time.

With what we've discussed so far in mind, let's now discuss the specific essential oils that you can use to deal with various problems such as stress, anxiety, and insomnia. In the following sections, we shall study various oils, their innate properties, and then learn how to blend or mix them with other effective oils.

To make the next section easier to understand, we will classify the oils based on the recommended application method.

Essential Oil Recipes for Stress Relief

The following essential oil blends will prove very effective to the treatment of stress.

1. DIY Stress-Reducing Solution

Ingredients

10 drops of myrrh EO

10 drops of lavender EO

10 drops of frankincense EO

10 drops of bergamot EO

Directions

In a dark colored glass bottle, add all the essential oils (the dark bottle helps reduce exposure to strong sunlight that can breakdown the oil).

Get a vertical dropper to help you control the amount of oil you use; you will need about 10 to 15 drops of the above blend mixed with a cup of Epsom salt in the bath.

Now secure the dispenser into the bottle and cap it. Shake to blend the oils then add 10-15 drops of the blend to Epsom salt if you intend to use the blend for hydrotherapy.

To diffuse the blend, fill your diffuser with water (or follow manufacturer's instructions), add 5-6 drops of the blend to the diffuser, and the place it in an area that allows the diffused mist to permeate every area of the room.

2. DIY Essential Oil Blend

Ingredients

20 drops of bergamot essential oil

30 drops of ylang ylang essential oil

25 drops of lavender essential oil

30 drops of cedar wood essential oil

20 drops of patchouli essential oil

Dark glass dropper bottle

Jojoba oil (optional)

Directions

Mix the essential oils in a glass dropper bottle or glass vial.

Dilute the essential oils blend with jojoba oil then run a few drops between your palms.

Deeply breathe in the scent to achieve an instant calming effect against stress and anxiety.

You can also add a few drops to a warm bath for a stress-fighting bath or add a few drops to your favorite moisturizer.

Mix with 1 part plain witch hazel and 1 part water. Add to a spray bottle to make a room spray.

3. Stress Relief Lotion

Ingredients

4 drops of Cedarwood (Atlas) essential oil

5 drops of clary sage essential oil

7 drops of grapefruit essential oil

24 drops of lavender essential oil

8 grams of emulsifying wax NF

75 grams of distilled water

25 grams of oil

Directions

Add emulsifying wax NF and oil to a tin can or heatproof jar. Measure the water and magnesium oil (optional) into a 250 milliliters canning jar.

Put both containers in a saucepan that has 1-2 inches of water. Set the pan on medium-low heat for around 10 minutes, and then pour the hot contents of the two cans together to create a milky-looking mixture.

At this point, briskly stir the lotion using a small whisk or fork for 30 to 45 minutes. Set aside to cool while stirring occasionally after every 30 seconds.

You can place the bowl with the mixture in a bowl of cold water to speed up the cooling process as the lotion thickens.

Now stir in essential oils and pour the lotion into a pump-top glass bottle. The lotion should thicken up within several hours or overnight.

Store the lotion for up to a week. To lengthen shelf-life, add a preservative such as 4 grams Leucidal Liquid SF.

4. Stress Reduction Inhaler

Ingredients

1 drop of chamomile essential oil

1 drop of geranium essential oil

4 drops of orange essential oil

4 drops of lavender essential oil

10 drops of bergamot essential oil

Directions

Measure a teaspoon of course salt and add it to a PET plastic bottle or dark glass bottle (go with the latter).

Add in the essential oils and shake to combine.

To use, take 3-4 long and deep breaths of the aroma. Take a short break then take another 3-4 breaths.

Administer the inhaler 3 times a day for optimal stress relieve.

5. Stress Relief Massage Oil

Ingredients

2 drops of petitgrain essential oil

1 drop of ylang ylang essential oil

5 drops of vegetable oil

2 drops of lavender essential oil

Directions

Add the essential oils along with carrier oil of choice in a glass container.

Stir to incorporate and then gently massage onto the body.

6. Uplifting Personal Blend

Ingredients

2 drops of rosewood essential oil

2 drops of geranium essential oil

2 drops of bergamot essential oil

Directions

In a container, combine 6 teaspoons of vegetable oil, 2 drops of bergamot oil, 2 drops of rosewood, and 2 drops geranium essential oils.

Use the blend by either inhaling directly from the bottle or massaging on the body during daytime.

7. Nighttime Uplifting Personal Blend

Ingredients

2 drops of Ylang Ylang essential oil

2 drops of HoWood essential oil

2 drops of bergamot essential oil

Directions

Add 6 drops of carrier oil to 2 drops of Ylang Ylang, 2 drops bergamot, and 1 drop HoWood essential oil.

Use the nighttime blend by massaging it on your body or inhaling directly from the bottle.

8. Stress-Relieving Blend 1

Ingredients

5 drops of Cedarwood essential oil

8 drops of Eucalyptus Globulus essential oil

12 drops of Lavender essential oil

12 drops of Geranium essential oil

18 drops of Marjoram essential oil

Directions

Combine the essential oils.

Rub the blend around your sinus passage or under your nose to help reduce stress and anxiety symptoms.

You can also massage the blend into the upper chest, along the back, on shoulders, and back of the neck before you sleep.

9. Stress-Relieving Blend 2

Ingredients

2 ounces of vegetable oil

1 drop of cardamom essential oil

1 drop of cinnamon leaf essential oil

2 drops of peppermint essential oil

2 drops of eucalyptus essential oil

8 drops of lemon essential oil

Directions

Combine the essential oils in a dark-colored bottle.

To use, add 2 teaspoons to your bath and use as massage oil or try 1 teaspoon for a footbath.

You can omit the carrier oil and diffuse into a diffuser or add 2 ounces of water to create an air spray.

Look for the package directions from the manufacturer of the air diffuser then add a few drops of your essential oil blend to make an effective blend. Use as desired.

10. Other Blends

Ingredients

4 drops of eucalyptus essential oil, 4 drops of spearmint essential oil, and 1 ounce of carrier oil

8 drops of lavender essential oil, 4 drops spearmint essential oil, and 1 ounce of carrier oil

4 drops or Roman chamomile essential oil, 8 drops of lavender essential oil, and 1 ounce of carrier oil

8 drops of lavender essential oil, 4 drops of spearmint essential oil, and 1 ounce of carrier oil

Directions

To make various blends, combine these oils and then dab a little amount to apply as required.

Try deeply massaging the blend onto your skin deeply for around 30 minutes, preferably a few minutes before you get under the covers for a restful night's sleep.

You can also use a diffuser to disperse the essential oil blend into the surrounding air, and then inhale the scented oils.

11. "It Is Well With My Soul" Blend

Ingredients

2 drops of cypress essential oil

2 drops of patchouli essential oil

2 drops of bergamot essential oil

Directions

Mix the patchouli oil, cypress and bergamot essential oils in a container.

Add suitable carrier oil such as jojoba or sweet almond oil.

Massage topically on the skin to relieve stress.

12. "Take It Easy" Diffuser Blend

Ingredients

1 drop of ylang ylang essential oil

1 drop of wild orange essential oil

1 drop of Cedarwood essential oil

3 drops of lavender essential oil

Directions

In a glass bottle, add all the essential oils along with carrier oil such as almond or jojoba vegetable oil.

Add the blend to a diffuser to melt all the worries and stresses of life away.

13. "Coastal Waters" Diffuser Blend

Ingredients

2 drops frankincense essential oil

2 drops orange essential oil

2 drops Cedarwood essential oil

1 drop rosemary essential oil

Directions

In a glass bowl or container, add in 2 drops of frankincense, 1 drop of rosemary oil, 2 drops of orange oil, and 2 drops of Cedarwood essential oils

To use the diffuser blend, follow the manufacturer's directions to add to the diffuser.

Place the diffuser at a strategic location where you can be inhaling the stress-relieving scent.

14. "Stress Less" Diffuser Blend

Ingredients

1 drop of marjoram essential oil

1 drop of ylang ylang essential oil

2 drops of clary sage essential oil

3 drops of lavender essential oil

Directions

Combine 1 drop of marjoram oil with a drop of ylang ylang, 2 drops of sage, and 3 drops of lavender essential oil

Add the mixture to a diffuser and inhale as desired.

15. "Refresh" Diffuser Blend

Ingredients

2 drops lime EO

2 drops bergamot EO

2 drops grapefruit EO

2 drops sandalwood EO

Directions

Combine 2 drops of sandalwood oil, 2 of drops lime oil, 2 of drops bergamot oil, and 2 drops grapefruit EO in a bottle.

Add the mixture to a diffuser or spray bottle and inhale as required.

Essential Oil Recipes That Enhance Relaxation

The following essential oil blends will help you relax:

16. Calming and Relaxing Blend

Ingredients

5 drops of lavender EO

10 drops Roman chamomile EO

1 ounce of sweet almond or other carrier oil

Directions

In an airtight container, mix all the essential oils and shake to incorporate.

Massage the blend onto various parts such as the feet.

To make a diffuser blend, just mix a drop of lavender with 2 drops of roman chamomile essential oil.

17. Daily Calming Blend

Ingredients

1 ounce of St. John's Wort essential oil

2 drops of frankincense essential oil

3 drops of German chamomile essential oil

3 drops of myrtle essential oil

6 drops of cypress essential oil

Directions

Mix the oils in a glass or plastic bottle.

Once well incorporated, apply topically on the skin through body massage.

Alternatively, you can prepare a salve by heating ½ teaspoon of shaved beeswax and then add the essential oils.

Dilute these oils with carrier oils such as avocado, sweet almond, or jojoba oil and then apply topically on the skin.

Simply combine an ounce of carrier oil with recommended drops of each essential oil to prepare a daily massage formula.

18. Pain-Relieving Blend

Ingredients

1 drop of peppermint essential oil

1 drop of clove essential oil

1 drop of calendula or chamomile essential oil

5ml of carrier oil

Directions

Combine the essential oils and then gently massage on the stomach in a clockwise motion.

19. Fatigue-Fighting Blend

Ingredients

2 drops of eucalyptus EO

2 ounces of vegetable oil

1 drop of cardamom EO

1 drop of cinnamon leaf EO

2 drops of peppermint EO

8 drops of lemon EO

Directions

Mix the essential oils in a dark-colored glass or plastic bottle.

Add 2 teaspoons of this blend to your bath or use as massage oil. If you need a footbath, try adding 1 teaspoon of the blend to water.

Try omitting the carrier oil if you want to use in an inhaler or diffuser.

Alternatively, add the blend to 2 ounces of water to create an air spray. Use as desired.

20. 3-Ingredient Relaxing Blend

Ingredients

1 tablespoon of vegetable oil

3 drops of tea tree essential oil

3 drops of lavender essential oil

Directions

Combine these essential oils in a suitable bottle, then rub around the face, and down along your lymph nodes (these are on the side of your neck).

You can also create a warm compress then place it over various body parts. For kids, use half of the amount to massage the body, preferably 2-3 times daily.

21. Healing and Relaxing Recipe

Ingredients

1 drop of rosemary EO

2 drops of eucalyptus EO

1 drop of black pepper EO

2 drops of peppermint EO

2 drops of lavender EO

15 ml of evening primrose oil

1 drop of tea tree EO

Directions

Prepare massage oil by combining the essential oils in a dark-colored glass bottle.

Shake well then rub the blend onto your temples, top of hands, back of the neck, or at the soles of the feet.

22. Aromatic Compress Blend

Ingredients

3 drops of lavender essential oil

1 drop of eucalyptus essential oil

1 cup of ice water

Directions

Combine the essential oils and the ice cold water in a bowl or bottle.

Swish to combine the oils and then soak a washcloth into the mixture.

Wring, place it on the forehead, and then repeat the process a couple of times while the mixture is still warm

You can also try making an aromatic sponging blend by adding 2 drops of chamomile oil to a basin of tepid water.

Simply fill your basin with water, add chamomile, and then soak a sponge into the water.

If using the relaxing blend on your kid, just lay a child on a towel and massage from the neck down as needed.

23. Post Workout Muscle Massage Blend

Ingredients

1oz. of jojoba essential oil

1oz. of organic sweet almond essential oil

3 drops of ginger essential oil

4 drops of cinnamon cassia essential oil

3 drops of chamomile essential oil

Directions

In a glass bottle, add all the essential oils along with almond or jojoba vegetable oils.

To use the blend, gently massage it on tense muscles particularly after a workout.

24. Soothing Muscle Massage Oil

Ingredients

1-ounce amber glass bottles with dropper

1 ounce of jojoba oil or other vegetable oil

4 drops Cedarwood essential oil

4 drops of basil essential oil

8 drops of spike lavender essential oil

8 drops of chamomile essential oil

Directions

Obtain a glass spray bottle with a dropper then fill it halfway with a vegetable oil of choice such as jojoba oil.

Add in the essential oils and fill the remaining space with the vegetable or carrier oil.

Tightly close the lid in place then properly swirl to incorporate the oils.

Gently drip the essential oil blend on sore areas and massage. Shake the bottle before each use.

25. Calming Sugar Body Scrub

Ingredients

2 tablespoons of certified organic argan essential oil

20 drops lavender essential oil

1 teaspoon of organic rose hip seed essential oil

4 tablespoon of organic turbinado sugar

Directions

Mix all the ingredients in a glass container and shake to combine.

To use the blend, rub the relaxing scrub onto the skin in circular motion.

Once done with exfoliating, rinse off.

26. Soothing Tea Time Bath

Ingredients

5 drops of chamomile essential oil or 5 drops peppermint essential oil

10-15 drops of Lavender essential oil

½ cup of dried lavender or chamomile flowers

¼ cup of baking soda

¼ cup of sea salt

¾ cup of Epsom salt or magnesium flakes

Directions

In a glass bowl or container, add all the dry ingredients and mix well.

Add in the essential oils and use a spoon to mix well. Take care not to touch the oils.

Use a spoon to fill each tea bag with the ingredients and draw the string tight.

To use, just run a warm bath and drop a few tea bags into the water while running. Keep the teabags in the water throughout the bath.

Once done with bathing, discard the tea bags.

27. Relaxation Massage Oil

Ingredients

1 drop of Frankincense essential oil

1 drop of Petitgrain essential oil

4 drops of Lavender essential oil

1 teaspoon of carrier oil/massage base

Directions

Add all the essential oils to a container along with 6 teaspoons of massage base.

Add the blend to a warm bath or use for a massage.

28. Balancing Perfume Blend

Ingredients

1 drop of bergamot essential oil

1 drop of copaiba essential oil

2 drops of frankincense essential oil

3 drops of grapefruit essential oil

1 tablespoon of fractionated coconut oil

1 dark glass roll-on bottle

Directions

Add all the essential oils in a roll-on bottle then fill the remaining capacity of the bottle with vegetable oil such as coconut oil.

Seal the bottle and store it in a dark place away from direct sunlight.

To use the oil blend, just massage to pulse points as required.

29. Invigorating Cologne

Ingredients

3 drops of Cedarwood essential oil

3 drops of Balsam Fir essential oil

1 tablespoon of fractionated coconut oil

1 dark glass roll-on bottle

Directions

Add all the essential oils in a roll-on bottle then fill the remaining capacity of the bottle with vegetable oil such as coconut oil.

Seal the bottle and store it in a dark place away from direct sunlight.

To use the oil blend, just massage on pulse points as required.

30. Muscle Love Bath Salts

Ingredients

1 cup of Epsom salt

5 drops of copaiba essential oil

10 drops of aroma siez essential oil

White lids

8-ounce glass pot

Directions

In a big glass bowl, mix the Epsom salt along with other essential oils.

Mix well using a metal spoon then pour the mixture into an 8-ounce glass pot and tightly cover with a lid.

To use, simply scoop out about ¼ or ½ cup of the blend and add to your bath.

31. Blend for Stress Relief

Ingredients

1 drop Ylang Ylang oil

2 drops Geranium oil

2 drops Clary Sage oil

3 drops Lavender oil

4 drops Roman Chamomile oil

Directions

Mix together the essential oils in a bowl or container. Shake to blend then add to your diffuser. Use as required to help you wind down and relax.

32. Mental Clarity Blend

Ingredients

1 drop of hyssop oil

1 drop of rosemary oil

1 drop of lemon oil

1 drop of peppermint oil

Directions

Mix together the essential oils above to create a perfect blend.

Add to your diffuser to help you boost concentration and your memory.

33. The Focus Blend

Ingredients

4 drops of doTERRA Balance

2 drops Vetiver oil

2 drops Frankincense oil

Directions

Combine the following oils in a bowl then add to your diffuser.

Place near your bed or other strategic place for easier diffusion.

Essential Oil Recipes For Improved Sleep

The following essential oil blends will improve your sleep:

34. Insomnia Blend

Ingredients

4 ounces of vegetable oil

2 drops of ylang ylang essential oil

3 drops of frankincense essential oil

10 drops of sandalwood essential oil

10 drops of lavender essential oil

15 drops of bergamot essential oil

Directions

Obtain the above oils. Combine them in a bottle and then massage into the skin or add 2 teaspoons into bath water.

To use into a diffuser, skip the vegetable oil and pour the mixture onto a potpourri cooker or a simmering pan of water and breathe into the fumes before going to bed preferably daily or until your sleeping patterns improves.

35. DIY Sleep Aid

Ingredients

Small dark-colored bottle with a tight lid

Diffuser

20 drops of bergamot essential oil

20 drops of Cedarwood essential oil

20 drops of frankincense essential oil

20 drops of lavender essential oil

Directions

In a small dark-colored glass or plastic bottle, combine all the essential oils and cap tightly.

Shake well to blend and set aside.

Add water to the diffuser based on the manufacturer's directions.

Add around 10 drops of the essential oil blend to the diffuser and place it at a strategic place point to ensure the diffused air fully permeates the room.

Turn it on when ready to use in your bedroom a few minutes before sleeping.

36. Peaceful Sleep Essential Oil Blend

Ingredients

1 drop of clary sage essential oil

3 drops of Lavender essential oil

1 teaspoon of cream

Directions

In a container, mix a drop of clary sage and 3 drops of lavender along with a teaspoon of cream of milk.

Now add this mixture to a warm bath and soak.

37. Peaceful Sleep Body Butter

Ingredients

7 ounces of liquid coconut oil

7 ounces of pure cocoa butter

7 ounces of organic Shea butter

7 ounces of coconut oil

<u>Peaceful Sleep Oil Blend</u>

Directions

Mix the coconut oil, Shea butter, and cocoa butter in a double boiler or microwave in a glass bottle or container.

Add in carrier oil of choice such as coconut oil then toss to combine.

Let the mixture cool for about 1 hour until it hardens, or instead, place the mixture in the fridge to accelerate the process.

As soon as the mixture sets, add a few drops of favorite your "<u>sleep essential oil blend</u>" based on the intensity of desired scent.

At this point, whip the body butter to achieve a nice fluffy texture; it should take about 10 minutes.

Drain the body butter into glass jars and then tightly seal each jar. To use the butter, just spread on the skin preferably before bed.

38. Sleep Tight Baby & Kids Blend

Ingredients

8 drops of vanilla essential oil

4 drops of lavender essential oil

Directions

Mix all the ingredients in a glass bowl or container.

To use, gently massage the baby on non-sensitive areas of the body.

39. Don't Snore Sleep Blend

Ingredients

1 drop of frankincense EO

2 drops of eucalyptus EO

2 drops of Cedarwood EO

5 drops of marjoram EO

5 drops geranium EO

5 drops of lavender EO

Directions

Mix the essential oils in a glass container.

To use, you can inhale a few drops of the blend or add to your diffuser.

Essential oils such as frankincense, Cedarwood, and lavender are helpful for snorers who have allergies or nasal congestion.

40. "Calm Me Down" Sleep Aid

Ingredients

5 drops of wild orange essential oil

5 drops of rosemary essential oil

10 drops of frankincense essential oil

Directions

Mix the frankincense, rosemary, and wild orange essential oils in a dark-colored glass bottle.

Add to your diffuser or massage with the blend a few minutes before bed. This blend is effective for insomnia related to anxiety.

41. "Restful Slumber" Blend

Ingredients

5 drops of Neroli EO

10 drops of lavender EO

5 drops of Cedarwood EO

Directions

Mix 10 drops of lavender, 5 drops of Cedarwood, and 5 drops Neroli essential oils in a bowl.

Add to the diffuser or use the blend for massage to promote the quality of sleep since Cedarwood promotes restful sleep.

42. "Make Me Sleepy" Diffuser Blend

Ingredients

5 drops of bergamot essential oil

5 drops of clary sage essential oil

10 drops of Roman chamomile essential oil

Directions

Combine the roman chamomile oil, clary sage, and bergamot essential oils in a glass container.

Apply 30-45 minutes before sleep to obtain or fall asleep easily. Clary sage is a sedative that helps calm your troubled mind.

43. Calming Blend for Sleep

Ingredients

5 drops of ylang ylang essential oil

10 drops of Roman chamomile essential oil

5 drops of lavender essential oil

Directions

Mix the lavender, roman chamomile, and Ylang Ylang essential oils in a container or bowl

Use the blend a few minutes before bed. Roman chamomile helps calm a racing mind and makes falling asleep easier.

44. Sleep Diffuser Blend 1

Ingredients

3 drops of Vetiver EO

3 drops of lavender EO

Few drops carrier oil of choice

2 drops of frankincense EO

Directions

In a glass bottle, add all the essential oils along with carrier oil such as almond or jojoba vegetable oil.

To use the blend, gently massage the blend on tense muscles particularly after a workout.

45. Sleep Diffuser Blend 2

Ingredients

2 drops of wild (sweet) orange EO

3 drops of patchouli EO

2 drops of frankincense EO

Few drops carrier oil of choice

Directions

Mix 3 drops of patchouli essential oil, 2 drops of orange essential oil, and 2 drops of frankincense in a dark bottle or container.

Shake to blend then massage or add to the diffuser few minutes before bed.

46. Sleep Diffuser Blend 3

Ingredients

2 drops of marjoram essential oil

2 drops of Roman chamomile essential oil

2 drops of lavender essential oil

Few drops carrier oil of choice

Directions

Mix the essential oils in a bottle then store in a cool and dark place.

Use it before bedtime to boost sleep quality. You can massage, inhale a few drops, or add to your bath.

You can add a carrier oil of choice to dilute the oils.

47. Sleep Diffuser Blend 4

Ingredients

2 drops of Roman chamomile essential oil

2 drops of lavender essential oil

3 drops of grounding blend essential oil

Few drops carrier oil of choice

Directions

Mix the essential oils in a dark-colored glass or plastic bottle.

Add 2 teaspoons of this blend to your bath or use as massage oil. If you need a footbath, try adding 1 teaspoon of the blend to water.

To use in an inhaler or diffuser, omit the carrier oil.

Alternatively, add 2 ounces of water and create an air spray. Use as desired.

48. Sleep Diffuser Blend 5

Ingredients

2 drops of frankincense essential oil

2 drops of bergamot essential oil

3 drops of Roman chamomile essential oil

Few drops carrier oil of choice

Directions

Mix the essential oils along with carrier oil of choice in a glass container.

Stir to incorporate then gently massage onto the body.

49. Relaxation & Sleep Blend

Ingredients

2 drops orange essential oil

2 drops marjoram oil

2 drops lavender oil

1 drop Roman chamomile oil

1 drop German chamomile oil

Directions

Mix together the following essential oils in a glass bowl or container.

Add to your diffuser by following its manufacturer's directions. Use or inhale as required.

50. Great Relaxer and Soother

Ingredients

2 drops Sandalwood essential oil

4 drops Ginger oil

6 drops lime oil

6 drops bergamot oil

6 drops grapefruit oil

Directions

Combine the suggested drops of each essential oil in a glass bowl.

Add the blend to your diffuser and place it at strategic position.

Conclusion

We have come to the end of the book. Thank you for reading and congratulations for reading until the end.

As you have seen, there are many applications of essential oils in addition to their refreshing scents. It's now your time to try most of these healing recipes from Mother Nature's gift of pure and therapeutic-grade oils.

Finally, if you found the book valuable, please take the time to share your thoughts and post a review on Amazon. It'd be greatly appreciated!

Thank you and good luck!